ACL RECONSTRUCTION SURGERY DIET

Unlocking The Power Of Nutrition And Fueling Recovery For Knee Joint Healing And Regaining Strength

DR LUCAS KAYCE

DISCLAIMER

This book about illness and nutrition is not meant to replace expert medical advice, diagnosis, or treatment; rather, it is meant purely for informational reasons. This book's content is founded on broad concepts and recommendations for managing diseases and nutrition.

Before adopting any major dietary or lifestyle changes, readers are recommended to speak with a qualified healthcare provider, such as a licensed physician or registered dietitian, especially if they have pre-existing medical concerns. Everybody has different health demands, so what works for one person might not work for another.

The use of the information provided in this book may have unfavorable repercussions or consequences, for which the author and publisher disclaim all liability. No disease is meant to be identified, treated, cured, or prevented by the information provided.

The book may include contain references to medical literature or research findings; however readers are urged to independently confirm this material and contact reliable sources.

It is important to remember that the fields of nutrition and medicine are always changing, and that new findings could have an impact on the advice offered in this book. As a result, readers are urged to keep up with the most recent advancements in healthcare and, when in doubt, seek professional counsel.

By reading this book, readers agree that they are in charge of their own health decisions and release the author and publisher from any liability arising from the use of the material in the book, whether direct or indirect.

TABLE OF CONTENTS

ABOUT THE BOOK

The book "ACL Reconstruction Surgery Diet" is a thorough manual that focuses on nutrition, which is a crucial part of the healing process following surgery. Recognizing the complex interplay between nutrition and healing, the book explores the role that dietary decisions play in maximizing the healing process following anterior cruciate ligament (ACL) reconstructive surgery.

The book give a basic overview of ACL reconstruction surgery, including topics such as preoperative planning, frequent injuries that result in reconstruction, and the anatomy of the ACL. These sections offer the groundwork for an in-depth examination of the critical function nutrition plays in the healing process. The main focus is on comprehending the subtleties of how diet affects inflammation, tissue healing, and total rehabilitation.

Beyond the theoretical, the book provides helpful advice in the form of postoperative and preoperative dietary suggestions. Along with specific food advice to speed up the healing process after surgery, readers are given practical methods to prepare their bodies for surgery. The use of vitamins and supplements as supportive measures gives the dietary approach a more comprehensive perspective.

One of the book's best features is the sample meal plans that are included for each stage of the recovery timetable. These meal plans provide readers with a practical guide on how to nourish their bodies at different phases of the rehabilitation process.

The book's dedication to diversity and adaptation is further evidenced by its special concerns, which include addressing dietary requirements, managing weight, and providing vegetarian and vegan options.

The book also expands on how nutrition relates to other aspects of recovery, such as exercise and rehabilitation. A well-rounded approach benefits from practical insights on increasing strength, integrating nutrition with physical therapy, and navigating the gradual return to physical activity.

 The book's section on mental and emotional wellness during rehabilitation captures its holistic approach. Understanding the complex relationship between diet and mental health, the book offers coping mechanisms and constructive thinking exercises to help readers maintain a positive outlook during their recovery.

The book offers advice on long-term nutritional considerations and upholding a healthy lifestyle, going beyond the short healing phase. Through its comprehensive coverage of the immediate as well as long-term issues of diet following ACL surgery, this book proves to be an invaluable tool for anybody navigating the intricacies of rehabilitation.

CHAPTER ONE

ACL RECONSTRUCTION SURGERY DIET OVERVIEW

In the fields of sports medicine and orthopedics, orthopedic procedures like Anterior Cruciate Ligament (ACL) reconstruction are becoming more and more common. The goal of anterior cruciate ligament restoration surgery is to restore a torn or injured anterior cruciate ligament, which is an essential stabilizing ligament in the knee joint. People who have suffered from sports-related injuries or other traumatic events that have resulted in ACL damage are frequently advised to have this surgery.

AN OVERVIEW OF SURGERY FOR ACL RECONSTRUCTION

The goal of ACL reconstruction surgery is to give the knee joint stability and functionality again through a precise and advanced process. The anterior cruciate ligament, which is found inside the knee, is essential for stability when performing actions like pivoting and jumping that require abrupt changes in direction. ACL injuries are frequent in sports like football, basketball, and soccer as well as in daily tasks involving quick, forceful movements.

During the procedure, a graft—usually an autograft from the patient's own body or an allograft from a donor—replaces the torn ACL. The patellar tendon, hamstring tendon, and quadriceps tendon are often utilized autografts. There are possibilities for cadaveric tissue allograft.

The surgeon's preference, the patient's age, and their degree of activity all influence the transplant selection.

A thorough rehabilitation program is necessary after surgery to maximize recovery. Restoring the knee's strength, range of motion, and functionality requires physical therapy. To give the graft time to integrate and the knee the opportunity to heal properly, patients are frequently recommended to avoid high-impact activities during the early phases of recovery.

DIET IS CRUCIAL TO THE HEALING PROCESS

The importance of a nutritious, well-balanced diet cannot be emphasized, even though surgery is an important first step on the road to recovery. During the rehabilitation phase, maintaining overall well-being, controlling inflammation, and assisting the healing process all depend on proper diet.

Tissue regeneration and repair require a diet high in vital nutrients such as proteins, vitamins, and minerals. For instance, proteins are essential for the manufacture of collagen, which is a vital constituent of tendons and ligaments. Lean proteins from foods such as fish, chicken, legumes, and dairy products can be incorporated to help rebuild tissues and muscle mass.

Vitamin C, vitamin D, and calcium are essential for the immune system and bone health in addition to proteins. The body uses these nutrients to maintain general strength and to heal damaged tissues. Staying properly hydrated is crucial for maintaining joint health and ensuring that body functions are operating at optimal capacity.

In addition, dietary considerations involve controlling body weight because being overweight can exacerbate the strain on the mending knee joint. Eating a well-balanced diet and getting enough calories helps you stay at a healthy weight and speed up your recuperation.

ACL restoration surgery is a complicated process that requires a multidisciplinary approach to healing. A healthy diet and a well-planned rehabilitation program are essential for maximizing results and guaranteeing a smooth transition back to regular activity. Understanding the significance of these interrelated components is essential to helping patients make a full recovery after ACL reconstruction surgery.

CHAPTER TWO

COMPREHENDING ACL RECONSTRUCTION SURGERY

THE ANTERIOR CRUCIATE LIGAMENT (ACL): WHAT IS IT?

The tibia (shinbone) and femur (thigh bone) should not move too much forward in respect to one another, which is prevented by the Anterior Cruciate Ligament (ACL), a vital ligament in the knee. Situated in the middle of the knee joint, this ligament is one of the four main ligaments in the body. When engaging in activities involving abrupt stops, direction changes, and pivoting, the ACL is crucial to maintaining optimal knee function.

THE REASONS AND TYPICAL INJURIES THAT LEAD TO ACL RECONSTRUCTION

ACL injuries are rather prevalent and can come from non-contact activities like abrupt direction changes, clumsy landings, or direct hits to the knee.

Sports requiring a lot of twisting, cutting, or jumping put athletes at higher risk of ACL damage. These injuries can vary in severity from partial tears to total ruptures, and they frequently cause a noticeable popping sound at the scene.

AN OVERVIEW OF SURGERY FOR ACL RECONSTRUCTION

ACL reconstruction surgery becomes a potential option when non-surgical treatments such as physical therapy and rehabilitation exercises are not enough to restore knee stability. The goal of ACL reconstruction surgery is to use a graft to repair the torn ligament.

The patient's patellar tendon, hamstring tendon, or cadaver (allograft) can all be used as sources for the graft. The surgeon's preference, the patient's age, and their level of activity all influence the graft selection.

The degree of instability felt, the activity level of the patient, and the severity of the injury all play a role in the decision to have ACL reconstruction surgery.

Persistent knee instability, trouble carrying out daily tasks, and a desire to resume sports or activities involving cutting, turning, and jumping are common reasons for surgery.

GETTING READY FOR SURGERY ON ACL RECONSTRUCTION

A thorough examination and planning procedure are necessary before having ACL restoration surgery. Pre-operative consultations, imaging tests, and talks on the actual surgical treatment may fall under this category. Prehabilitation, a type of pre-surgery rehabilitation, could be suggested in particular circumstances to strengthen the surrounding muscles and enhance the knee's general state before the procedure.

Patients are also asked to provide the surgical team with their full medical history, including any prescription drugs and dietary supplements they may be using. This information aids in evaluating the surgery's possible risks and complications. To make sure the patient is educated and at ease with the impending treatment, alternatives for anesthesia and possible post-operative care plans are also addressed during the preparation stage.

Comprehending ACL reconstruction surgery entails realizing the role of the Anterior Cruciate Ligament in knee stability, figuring out the typical reasons and injuries that necessitate reconstruction, and realizing the extensive process of getting ready for the procedure. After suffering a ligamentous injury to the knee, an important first step toward function restoration and resuming an active lifestyle is ACL reconstruction.

CHAPTER THREE

NUTRITION'S ROLE IN THE HEALING PROCESS

It is impossible to exaggerate the role that diet plays in the healing process. A diet that is high in nutrients and well-balanced is essential for promoting the body's ability to heal after a variety of ailments, operations, and injuries. The body often needs more food during the recovery period because it needs the extra energy and nutrients to repair damaged tissues and cells. Sufficient nourishment not only speeds up the healing process but also lowers the chance of problems and improves general health.

HOW NUTRITION IMPACTS HEALING AND INFLAMMATION

Food has a big influence on inflammation and how quickly the body heals. Extended recuperation periods may be caused by persistent inflammation, which can hinder the healing process.

A diet high in anti-inflammatory foods, such as fruits, vegetables, and omega-3 fatty acids, can help reduce inflammation and encourage a faster recovery. Conversely, some meals, like those high in refined sugars and saturated fats, can make inflammation worse.

ESSENTIAL NUTRIENTS FOR REPAIRING TISSUE

A complete recovery depends on the presence of several nutrients in the diet, as they are crucial for tissue regeneration. For example, protein is an essential component of tissues, muscles, and organs.

Consuming enough protein is essential for mending harmed tissues and encouraging the development of new, healthy cells. In addition, the synthesis of collagen and other substances necessary for wound healing and tissue regeneration depends on vitamins and minerals including copper, zinc, and A.

HYDRATION'S EFFECT ON REHABILITATION

One important element that has a big impact on the healing process is hydration. Maintaining appropriate body functions, such as waste disposal, temperature regulation, and nutrient transfer, depends on drinking enough water. Maintaining adequate hydration makes it more likely that nutrients will reach the healing process's participating cells effectively.

Being dehydrated increases the risk of problems and slows down the healing process by impairing blood circulation. Thus, it is crucial to keep the fluid balance appropriate to aid the body's healing processes.

Nutrition plays a variety of roles in recovery and is essential to the entire healing process. In addition to providing the energy needed, a healthy diet also delivers the vital elements needed for tissue regeneration and repair.

A well-planned diet that targets inflammation and has the proper ratio of proteins, vitamins, and minerals can make a big difference in how quickly and effectively someone recovers. Furthermore, maintaining optimal physiological functions that promote healing is essential for supporting the body's rehabilitation efforts. This can be achieved by drinking enough water.

CHAPTER FOUR

GUIDELINES FOR PREOPERATIVE NUTRITION

GUIDELINES FOR PREOPERATIVE NUTRITION

HOW TO GET YOUR BODY READY FOR SURGERY

It is important to properly prepare your body before surgery to improve general health and speed up the healing process. Preoperative preparation entails several activities, such as managing stress, optimizing diet, and adhering to particular recommendations made by medical experts. A faster recovery, fewer complications after surgery, and improved surgical outcomes can all be attributed to adequate planning.

RECOMMENDED DIET FOR PREOPERATIVE CARE

A healthy, well-balanced diet is essential for getting the body ready for surgery. Eating a diet high in vital nutrients—such as proteins, carbs, fats, vitamins, and minerals—is advised.

Protein is essential for the healing process following surgery because it plays a special role in immune system activity and tissue repair. Energy comes from carbohydrates, while healthy fats help absorb fat-soluble vitamins and maintain general cell function.

People are frequently told to concentrate on eating lean proteins like chicken, fish, tofu, and lentils in the days before surgery. To acquire a range of vitamins and minerals, you should also incorporate fruits, vegetables, and whole grains. Equally important is hydration, which patients should continue to consume in moderation to avoid dehydration, which can hinder their recuperation after surgery.

It's imperative to stay away from a few specific foods and drinks during the preoperative phase. Eating foods high in fat and grease might aggravate digestive issues and raise the possibility of surgical complications. Alcohol and caffeine should be used in moderation since they may interfere with anesthesia and cause dehydration.

VITAMINS & SUPPLEMENTS FOR SUPPORT BEFORE SURGERY

To promote optimal preoperative health, a balanced diet may be combined with recommendations for certain vitamins and supplements. Vitamin C can aid in the healing of wounds because of its function in the creation of collagen.

Blood clotting is dependent on vitamin K, which lowers the possibility of severe bleeding before and after surgery. For bone health, calcium and vitamin D are essential and may be advised, particularly for those who are deficient in these nutrients.

Fish oil supplements contain omega-3 fatty acids, which have anti-inflammatory qualities and may help the body heal from surgery-related stress.

Before starting any new supplements, it's crucial to speak with medical specialists because some supplements have the potential to interfere with prescriptions or affect the results of surgery.

Getting your body ready for surgery requires a multifaceted strategy that centers on a preoperative diet that is well-balanced and, if needed, vitamin and mineral supplementation. Consulting with medical professionals guarantees customized advice based on each patient's needs, which helps to maintain the best possible preoperative condition and fosters a positive surgery experience.

CHAPTER FIVE

GUIDELINES FOR POSTOPERATIVE NUTRITION

NEEDS FOR IMMEDIATE POSTOPERATIVE NUTRITION

For surgical patients' recovery and overall health, they require Immediate Postoperative Nutrition Needs. The body's metabolic needs frequently rise in the immediate post-operative period as it attempts to mend tissue damage and heal wounds. Consequently, to support the body's energy needs during this crucial phase, a well-planned and nutritionally balanced postoperative diet is crucial. Usually, patients are told to begin with foods that are simple to digest and supply vital nutrients without overtaxing their digestive systems.

USING DIET TO CONTROL PAIN AND INFLAMMATION

A crucial part of postoperative therapy is the Dietary Management of Pain and Inflammation. Some foods have anti-inflammatory qualities that can help lessen pain and inflammation. Walnuts, flaxseeds, and seafood all contain omega-3 fatty acids, which are well known for their anti-inflammatory properties. Consuming foods high in antioxidants, such as fruits and vegetables, can also aid in the fight against oxidative stress, which is frequently more intense in the aftermath of surgery. Modulating inflammation also requires a balanced ratio of omega-6 to omega-3 fatty acids, which can be maintained by limiting the amount of processed oils consumed.

THE FUNCTION OF PROTEIN IN MUSCLE REPAIR

After surgery, protein is essential for muscle recovery. Consuming enough protein is necessary for the creation of new tissues and the restoration of damaged cells. This is especially crucial for people who have had surgical operations that resulted in harm to the muscles or tissues. The postoperative diet should include high-quality protein sources such as lean meats, poultry, fish, eggs, and dairy products. To make sure patients get enough protein, particularly if their diet is limited, protein supplements could also be advised.

MINERALS AND VITAMINS FOR HEALING

Minerals and vitamins are essential for the recovery process following surgery. Tissue repair and wound healing are significantly aided by specific vitamins and minerals. For instance, the manufacture of collagen, a vital constituent of connective tissue, depends on vitamin C. Another micronutrient that boosts immunity and promotes wound healing is zinc. To guarantee that they obtain enough of the vital vitamins and minerals they need while recovering, patients are advised to eat a range of fruits, vegetables, whole grains, and lean proteins.

STRATEGIES FOR HYDRATION AFTER SURGERY

Hydration Techniques After Surgery: It's critical to maintain physiological processes, avoid dehydration, and help the body flush out waste. After surgery and anesthesia, it is even more important to drink enough fluids because these conditions might cause fluid loss. Although electrolyte-rich beverages may be advised, particularly if electrolyte imbalances are a concern, water is still the primary and recommended choice for hydration. Ensuring adequate hydration throughout the recovery phase requires monitoring urine production and being aware of indicators of dehydration, such as dark urine or dry mouth.

Postoperative nutrition is a complex area of patient care that includes managing pain and inflammation with food, meeting immediate nutritional needs, the role of vitamins and minerals in healing, the significance of protein in muscle recovery, and hydration techniques to promote general health. A nutrient-dense, well-balanced diet that is customized for each patient is essential for encouraging the best possible recovery and reducing postoperative problems.

CHAPTER SIX

EXAMPLE MENUS

EARLY POSTOPERATIVE DAYS

The main goal of meal plans in the immediate aftermath of surgery, particularly in the first few days following the procedure, is to promote the body's natural healing process and facilitate a speedy recovery. Patients may have decreased appetite and even stomach issues at this time. Thus, it's critical to give easy-to-digest and nutrient-dense diets priority. Clear liquids are vital for supplying necessary electrolytes and preventing dehydration. Examples of these include broths, clear soups, and herbal teas. It's usually advised to eat small, frequent meals that are high in protein and low in fat to support healing and sustain energy levels.

WEEKS 1-2 POST-SURGERY

More varied and textured foods are gradually introduced as patients go from the acute postoperative phase into the first two weeks of recuperation.

During this time, meal plans start to emphasize soft and readily digestible foods. Lean meats, eggs, and dairy products are good sources of protein, which is still necessary for tissue repair. Including a range of fruits and vegetables will also help supply vital vitamins and minerals, which can speed up the healing process overall. It's critical to stay hydrated and keep an eye out for any indications of food intolerance.

WEEKS 3–4 FOLLOWING SURGERY

Patients usually see an increase in their ability to tolerate a greater variety of foods by these weeks. Proteins, carbs, and healthy fats are among the macronutrients that should be included in a balanced diet plan at this stage. In terms of texture, the emphasis gradually moves from a diet that is mostly composed of soft meals to one that includes more fibrous and solid foods. Taking into account individual differences in appetite and digestion, portion control becomes crucial. It is advised that patients pay attention to their body's signals of hunger and fullness and modify them as necessary. It's still important to drink enough water to help the body repair and recuperate.

WEEKS 5-8 FOLLOWING SURGERY

Patients frequently report a marked improvement in their general state of well-being and a rise in energy during these weeks following surgery. During this stage, meal plans keep getting more creative and include a wider variety of foods and textures. The focus is on including nutrient-dense foods including whole grains, lean proteins, and a range of fruits and vegetables that promote long-term healing. Individual exercise levels and any special dietary recommendations made by medical professionals may also influence portion sizes. As the body continues to rebuild strength, this phase represents an important shift toward a more consistent and long-lasting feeding pattern.

Long-Term Recovery Meal Plans: The goal of long-term recovery meal plans is to create dietary habits that are both healthful and sustainable, supporting long-term well-being.

Returning to a more typical diet during this phase is important, with a focus on consuming nutrients in balance. These meal plans are built on a foundation of whole grains, lean proteins, healthy fats, and an assortment of fruits and vegetables. Portion control and taking into account any long-term dietary limitations or advice from medical professionals is still crucial. To support ongoing healing and general health, patients are advised to pay attention to their bodies, make educated dietary choices, and prioritize eating a well-rounded diet. Frequent check-ups with medical professionals can aid in fine-tuning dietary regimens according to each person's requirements and advancement.

CHAPTER SEVEN

PARTICULAR POINTS TO REMEMBER

VEGETARIAN AND VEGAN OPTIONS

Taking dietary preferences and limits into account has grown in importance in the field of special considerations, with a particular emphasis on vegetarian and vegan lifestyles. These decisions are frequently motivated by moral, environmental, or health considerations.

It is important to consider providing a variety of enticing options for people who follow different dietary pathways when organizing meals or celebrations. Meat is not allowed in vegetarianism, but veganism goes a step further and forbids the consumption of any animal products, including dairy and eggs.

Event planners, eateries, and rehab centers should make sure there is a wide selection of nutrient-dense substitutes to accommodate the needs of vegetarians and vegans.

This can entail adding plant-based proteins to diets, such as quinoa, lentils, and tofu. Furthermore, providing a variety of vibrant fruits, veggies, and whole grains improves the nutritional content and fosters a more welcoming dining environment.

Everyone may have a well-rounded and fulfilling culinary experience when vegetarian and vegan dishes are thoughtfully and creatively prepared.

MANAGING WEIGHT DURING RECOVERY

Keeping a healthy weight is a complex issue that requires close consideration of one's physical and emotional health.

People recovering from surgeries or eating problems, for example, frequently encounter particular difficulties keeping their weight in check. Beyond just a number on a scale, the emphasis should be on a comprehensive strategy that takes into account dietary requirements, psychological aspects, and general lifestyle.

It is crucial to include a balanced diet that takes into account dietary deficits. A customized meal plan can assist people in meeting their calorie and nutrient needs. It is created in partnership with nutritionists and healthcare providers. Lean proteins, whole grains, fruits, and vegetables may all be included in this. In addition, encouraging mindful eating and developing a healthy connection with food are crucial elements of managing weight while recovering from an eating disorder. Maintaining a healthy weight over time requires finding a balance between exercise and rest that is specific to each person's needs.

HANDLING DIETARY RESTRICTIONS AND ALLERGIES

In a variety of contexts, including hospitality and healthcare, understanding and accommodating dietary restrictions and allergies has become essential. To protect their safety and well-being, those with allergies or particular dietary requirements need to be treated with extra care.

Considering the seriousness of allergies to common foods like shellfish, dairy, nuts, or gluten, event planners and food service providers must establish comprehensive precautions.

Individuals with dietary limitations and the appropriate specialists must collaborate and communicate in detail. To provide a safe workplace, it is essential to have knowledgeable staff members, clearly labeled ingredients, and effective communication routes for dietary preferences. One of the most important aspects of inclusive hospitality is creating menus that cater to certain allergies or dietary requirements without sacrificing flavor or diversity. Businesses and institutions can create an atmosphere where people with dietary restrictions can comfortably participate in social and communal activities without sacrificing their health and well-being by giving priority to these considerations.

CHAPTER EIGHT

PHYSICAL ACTIVITY AND RECOVERY

COMBINING PHYSICAL THERAPY WITH DIET

Combining nutrition and physical therapy is a comprehensive strategy meant to maximize the general health and recuperation of patients receiving treatment. A balanced diet should be followed in addition to therapeutic measures since more and more medical practitioners are realizing the connection between physical health and nutrition. In the treatment of ailments including musculoskeletal injuries, chronic pain, and post-surgical rehabilitation, this integration is very important.

A carefully thought-out dietary plan supplies the vital nutrients required for muscle rehabilitation, tissue repair, and general healing, which enhances the objectives of physical therapy. The body needs proteins, carbs, lipids, vitamins, and minerals to sustain its physiological processes.

These nutrients also help make rehabilitation programs more successful. A thorough rehabilitation strategy must include nutrition consultations and dietary assessments to guarantee that patients receive individualized assistance to fulfill their specific nutritional demands.

NUTRITION TO DEVELOP POWER AND STURDINESS

Exercise and rehabilitation have as their primary goals the development of strength and endurance, and nutrition is essential to reaching these ends. To meet the demands of increased physical activity, muscle growth, and cardiovascular health, a nutrient-rich diet is necessary. For the synthesis of muscle proteins, which aid in the maintenance and growth of lean muscle mass, an adequate protein diet is essential. As the body's main energy source, carbohydrates support the resupply of glycogen and power physical activity.

Furthermore, incorporating healthy fats into the diet in a deliberate manner promotes overall energy balance and facilitates the absorption of fat-soluble vitamins. Iron and vitamin D are two examples of micronutrients that are essential for sustaining normal physiological processes and avoiding deficits that might hamper the development of strength and endurance training. As adequate fluid intake affects thermoregulation, joint lubrication, and overall exercise performance, hydration is equally important.

RETURNING TO PHYSICAL ACTIVITY GRADUALLY:

A key component of rehabilitation is the idea of a gradual return to physical activity, which guarantees a secure and long-lasting transition for people healing from illnesses or accidents.

This method recognizes the value of gradually exposing the body to workouts and activities so that it can adjust and rebuild strength without running the danger of re-injury or setbacks. Physical therapists take great care when creating graded exercise plans, taking into account each person's unique condition, functional limitations, and general level of fitness.

A staged approach that begins with low-intensity exercises and progresses to more difficult activities is what is meant by a gradual return to physical activity. This helps with psychological issues as well as physical healing, boosting self-esteem and lowering the fear of getting hurt again. It's critical to track the patient's reaction to each stage so that therapists may customize the rehabilitation plan and make any necessary modifications. A complete and personalized approach to the progressive return to physical activity is made possible by collaborative communication between patients, healthcare experts, and fitness trainers, when relevant. This ensures long-lasting improvements in health and functionality.

CHAPTER NINE

PAST RECUPERATION,

LONG-TERM FOOD RECOMMENDATIONS

When it comes to long-term nutritional considerations, sustainable and healthy practices are prioritized over fleeting fad diets and restrictive eating patterns. The foundation of a comprehensive strategy is knowledge of the body's long-term dietary requirements.

It entails developing a more thoughtful and harmonious connection with food than just tracking calories or following tight guidelines.

Realizing that every person is different and has different nutritional needs is an important part of long-term dietary planning. Since there isn't a single strategy that works for everyone, people are urged to experiment and find what suits their bodies the best. This means adjusting food choices to the body's cues, such as those of hunger and satiety.

Long-term health maintenance requires consuming a wide variety of nutrient-dense meals. A nourishing diet is built with an emphasis on complete, unprocessed foods such as fruits, vegetables, whole grains, lean proteins, and healthy fats. This method supports the body's numerous activities and not only gives vital vitamins and minerals, but also enhances general well-being.

The development of a flexible and happy attitude toward food is a crucial part of long-term dietary considerations. This entails giving up strict dietary guidelines and adopting a more instinctive eating style. Having a positive connection with food means experiencing meals guilt-free, cultivating a balanced mindset that allows for occasional indulgences without going against overall nutritional goals, and appreciating food.

Moreover, maintaining long-term nutritional success requires an awareness of the importance of hydration. Drinking enough water is essential for several body processes, such as digestion, absorption of nutrients, and control of body temperature. Including this knowledge in everyday activities enhances general health and supports other dietary decisions.

SUSTAINING AN INVIGORATING LIFESTYLE

A healthy lifestyle goes beyond eating; it's a comprehensive strategy that takes into account mental health, physical activity, and long-lasting behaviors. Frequent exercise supports cardiovascular health, muscular strength, and general energy, making it the cornerstone of a healthy lifestyle. Exercise that you love and can fit into your daily schedule is beneficial for your mental and emotional health in addition to your physical health.

Maintaining a healthy lifestyle requires not only physical exercise but also mental well-being. This entails using several stress-reduction strategies, such as mindfulness, meditation, or partaking in enjoyable and relaxing activities.

Maintaining a happy outlook and avoiding burnout requires striking a balance between work, play, and rest.

Sustaining general well-being also heavily depends on cultivating positive interpersonal interactions. Social ties boost one's sense of belonging, lessen feelings of loneliness, and offer emotional support. Whether they are with friends, family, or the community, fostering these relationships improves life quality and promotes emotional and mental toughness.

Sustainable practices that support a healthy lifestyle greatly include getting enough sleep and maintaining a regular sleep routine. Sleep affects immune system health, mood, and cognitive performance, making it a vital component of overall well-being. To be healthy in the long run, one must establish and stick to a schedule that places a high priority on getting enough sleep.

Leading a healthy lifestyle requires an all-encompassing, individualized strategy that incorporates sustainable habits, mindful eating, frequent exercise, and mental wellness.

CHAPTER TEN

EMOTIONAL AND MENTAL WELLBEING

NUTRITION'S FUNCTION IN MENTAL HEALTH

For mental health to be maintained and enhanced, proper nutrition is essential. There is a complex interplay between our mental health and our diet, with different nutrients having an impact on how the brain functions. Important nutrients include vitamins, minerals, amino acids, and omega-3 fatty acids help to produce neurotransmitters, which are chemical messengers that carry messages throughout the brain. For example, omega-3 fatty acids, which are present in walnuts, flaxseeds, and fish, are proven to boost brain health and may be beneficial for regulating mood.

Furthermore, a varied and balanced diet supplies the energy required for the best possible brain performance. Mood and cognitive performance can be impacted by blood sugar levels, which are controlled by the kinds and timing of meals.

Eating a diet rich in complex carbohydrates—like those found in whole grains and vegetables—helps control blood sugar levels and gives the brain a reliable source of energy. Conversely, consuming too many processed meals and refined sugars can cause blood sugar oscillations, which can affect mood swings and mental health in general.

Apart from nutrients, adequate water is essential for mental well-being. Dehydration can disrupt mood and emotional stability by impairing concentration and cognitive function. Maintaining optimal brain function and promoting emotional resilience requires drinking enough water.

HANDLING DIFFICULTIES WHILE RECOVERING

The road to recovery is paved with obstacles, and mastering useful coping skills is essential to getting through them. Developing a robust support network is a crucial component of coping during the healing process. Friends, family, or support groups are great places to find understanding and sympathetic people to lean on for emotional support and motivation. Building a sense of connection and understanding with people who have traveled similar paths can be facilitated by sharing experiences and difficulties.

During the rehabilitation process, self-awareness and mindfulness are effective coping mechanisms. People can become more conscious of their thoughts and emotions by practicing techniques like yoga, deep breathing exercises, and meditation. People with greater self-awareness are better able to recognize triggers, control stressors, and react to difficulties in a calm and collected way.

Another essential component of coping during recovery is setting reasonable goals and acknowledging minor accomplishments. By dividing more ambitious goals into smaller, more achievable ones, the trip becomes less daunting.

Acknowledging any kind of improvement, no matter how tiny gives one a sense of success and inspires them to keep going.

Getting professional assistance, like counseling or therapy, can also be a great way to get direction and support while going through the healing process. Counselors can help people explore underlying difficulties, create coping mechanisms, and strengthen their resilience. For continued improvement and mental health, it is crucial to acknowledge that setbacks are a normal part of the healing process and to learn from them.